Courage to Continue

Steps for Boldly Surmounting Life's Adversities

Dr. Ivan Hernandez

Strategic Book Publishing and Rights Co.

Strategic Book Publishing and Rights Co., LLC
USA | Singapore

For information about special discounts for bulk purchases, please contact Strategic Book Publishing and Rights Co. Special Sales, at bookorder@sbpra.net.

ISBN: 978-1-946539-19-9

Book Design: Suzanne Kelly
Cover Artwork: Keshuna Franklin
Photography: Keith Estep
Edited by: Casey Hynes

Dr. Ivan Hernandez is a father, doctor of physical therapy, fitness enthusiast, board certified orthopedic and sports clinician, movement expert, strength and conditioning specialist, and transformation coach.

Booking contact:

Dr. Syleecia Thompson
Dygmanagement@gmail.com

Dr. Ivan Hernandez on Social Media

Twitter: @DrIvanPT
Instagram: Dr.IvanPT
Facebook: DrIvanPT
Website: www.executiveparkpt.com

Dedication

I dedicate this book to my big brother, Ray. Despite being only two years older than me, I have always seen him as a much more mature person. He inspires many of my best decisions, from the coats we wore as children to the careers we pursued as adults. He is the shoulder on which I lean, my guardian angel, and my mentor, and I owe a great deal of my perseverance to him. Countless times he has given me the strength to endure the most difficult moments in my life. Ray has encountered the vicissitudes life throws at you in his own experiences, and witnessing his resilience has empowered me to remain strong and bolstered my ability to overcome my own challenges.

Table of Contents

Foreword

by Ray Hernandez

This book is the story of Ivan's life in his own words—his tribulations and his way of succeeding despite the trials. As Ivan's brother, I have had the privilege of witnessing his life as a journey through struggles and triumphs.

Ivan's story began thirty-nine years ago. We were born two years apart in the 1970s to a young Puerto Rican couple living in the South Bronx. Like many other kids coming up in the Bronx at that time, our family had limited resources. We were disenfranchised and exposed to violence, trauma, and painful domestic issues. Our lives progressed in a wayward motion, and for years we were unaware of what direction we would take. This was our status quo. We embraced the unpredictable nature of life by understanding that good times were measured by having our basic needs met for prolonged periods.

Most times, all Ivan and I had was each other. One of my earliest memories of Ivan took place when he was three years old. Even as a toddler, Ivan had an innate ability to see the world for what it was and how it could be made better. I can clearly remember Ivan being engrossed in playing with our action hero dolls. We had a collection of twelve-inch figurines that included Superman, Batman and Robin, Shazam, and Spiderman. We played with them for countless hours. On this particular day, one of Ivan's favorite doll's legs was pulled out of its socket. The toy was beyond repair. At least that's what I thought. Ivan, even at such an early age, took that doll with its amputated leg and taped the appendage to its body. Just like that, he restored its function. Ivan saved the superhero and went back to playing without another word.

That story is telling of Ivan's way of approaching dysfunction and integrating simple practical measures to restore, enhance, and promote well-being. No challenge has ever been too great for Ivan to surmount, despite the perils, dilemmas, tragedies, and catastrophic events he's encountered. Ivan has demonstrated throughout his life that through hard work, compassion, and integrity, one can find success, healing, and achievement.

Acknowledgments

I would be remiss if I began this book without sharing the driving force behind my resilience on this life journey — my two beautiful, intelligent, and caring boys, Ivan Jr. and Henry. They inspire me to go on even when I'm at rock bottom. If it were not for them, you would not be reading this book. Without them in my life, the climb out of the mental abyss that pulled me into its depths would have seemed insurmountable. They have kept me focused, busy, and full of laughter since they were born. They are my rocks, and I love them dearly.

My brother Ray, my guardian angel, has always brought clarity to my life, even during the cloudiest of times. He made sense of chaos and always assured me that even the worst wounds eventually heal. I will never forget his words: "You will develop a scar and will forever remember what caused it, but it will no longer hurt you the way it once did." He taught me that even vicissitudes have a purpose. He motivated me and emboldened me, and when I could not stand, he offered himself as my crutch. I will forever be indebted to the grace that he has laid upon my life. Ray helped me realize that even during the darkest of hours, there was something much larger at work, even if I could not see it at the time. He inspires me to fulfill every last inch of my potential.

My mother has always epitomized love and care in my eyes. As the mother of two young boys growing up in the sometimes rough world of the Bronx, she taught me the value of hard work and embodied endurance and mental toughness. She cared for Ray and me while working full-time and volunteering in the community, driven by her singular desire to create a good life and a promising future for her two sons. When I look back, I see the impression her unconditional love and perseverance made on me, even at a young age. Her example guides me now that I am a parent myself and understand what it is to want the world for my own two sons. Her comforting ways enabled me to stay strong throughout my life, especially during the journey I share in this book. I am the person I am today because of my mother's love, devotion, and inspirational character.

On paper, Cecilia Clement is my office manager. But she has really been a second mother to me. While proficient as a book-keeper and adept with managing multiple business egos, her best qualities are bringing people together and offering a firm and reassuring presence. When I think about her impact on my life and the many uplifting words that she has shared with me, nothing has resonated more than "Calm heads will always prevail." She has provided perspective and optimism as I weathered personal storms, and I will forever be indebted to her.

Many other people have played instrumental roles in guiding me out of the depths of adversity. From close friends to professional colleagues and team members, you know who you are and that you have become part of my family and my journey. I thank all of you, and I am eternally grateful for your tireless work on my behalf.

Last but certainly not least, I would be downright neglectful if I did not mention the person who made me face my fears for all the world to see, the person who saw something in me and promised to stand by my side as I worked toward the greatness she envisioned for me. She is meticulous, earnest, optimistic, caring, funny, and an all-around terrific person. In the past, I would have said that I met her coincidentally. I was in the market for an entertainment agent such as herself when she became a patient in my office. But I believe it was divine intervention that caused our paths to cross. For all she has done in my life, I vehemently exclaim my gratitude to Dr. Syleecia Thompson. Thank you for believing in me. I look forward to all our future prospects in the entertainment world.

CHAPTER ONE

Don't Judge a Book by Its Cover

*"Optimal wellness is more than skin
deep because what you see is not always
what you are."*

– Dr. Ivan Hernandez

I still remember exiting the ambulance on a gurney, clutching my chest in utter shock. I glimpsed my brother Ray making his way toward me as the medic rushed me through the doors of the ER. Ray was always there for me when I needed him the most. He's been my guardian angel throughout my life. Here he was again, his face full of concern, his body language suggesting that this was much more than the indigestion we had originally suspected. I had been sure the discomfort hardly merited attention until a cardiologist in the ER decided to do an echocardiogram. The test had immediately suggested a larger issue with my heart. There on the screen was the proof — part of my heart was damaged. The ER doctor turned to me and said, "You're having a heart attack."

It was all so surreal, and everything happened so quickly. I had barely registered the doctor's words before I was forced to make a fast decision: Did I want to be transferred to Columbia Presbyterian Hospital in New York City or stay locally at Lawrence Hospital in Bronxville, New York, to be treated? My thoughts ran wild. I wasn't prepared to have a heart attack. In fact, I woke up that morning anticipating a physically active day. What had gone wrong? How was this possible? I was young, active, and healthy. I ate well and exercised. To the outside observer, I was in top physical condition. However, I was also experiencing a great deal of stress, both personally and professionally. At first it rained, and then it poured, and now here I was lying on a gurney. The roof had collapsed and water had begun to flood the building.

Can it get any worse? I wondered. In a matter of months, I had been bombarded with problems that spiraled out of my control. In college, I studied psychology, and Abraham Maslow's hierarchy of needs concept always resonated with me. The basic premise is that to reach our full potential, we first must meet our basic needs. Things like sleep, a healthy diet, and love are critical to our survival. I followed this theory in all areas of my life because I knew that if I didn't take care of myself, it would be only a matter of time before my body succumbed to stress. To my mind, I did everything right. I practiced daily intermittent fasting, followed a modified Bulletproof diet, and incorporated a variety of lifting exercises in my workout regimen. Despite all of those efforts, my body succumbed anyway. I realized in the aftermath of my heart attack that I had neglected one of Maslow's most important needs — love.

My heart attack produced a pain I had never before experienced. It was deep and it was real. My body had been stricken with disease, but I didn't notice until it was almost too late because my emotional health was in even worse condition. A billow of dark clouds had settled over me when I woke the morning of my heart attack, and an indescribable solemnness settled in my soul. Years of suppressed pain exploded into this catastrophic event, sending me teetering on the edge between life and death. My ego had prevented me from registering the emotional pain I had experienced in early adulthood, and I pushed it deep down inside myself, thinking I could will it away. In the years immediately prior to my heart attack, I had become a walking zombie, going through the motions as a shell of my former self. On the surface, I lived an ideal existence. In reality, I wore a veil that concealed all that I wished to hide from the world.

The Day Before

I sat in my office dutifully typing my clinical notes, fatigued from a full day of seeing patients. It had been a busy but unremarkable day. No difficult patients, no conflicts, and no personal issues were bringing me down—at least no more than usual. Life had become challenging in recent months, but focusing on patients had given me a reprieve from my personal woes and even invigorated me for a time. I've always been one to consider the day a good one if I remained unscathed by the typical stress-provoking events that occur when working with a wide range of personalities, as one does in the medical field. The only thoughts on my mind that evening were of the mundane chores that awaited me at my apartment: cooking, cleaning, and preparing for the next day. I planned to finish my patients' charts, go home and marinate the chicken I had defrosted that morning, and then meet up with my neighbor, who happened to be my workout partner and a good friend. Both of us had taken to exercise as a way of bettering ourselves and a means to unload our daily stresses. We often pushed ourselves hard, incrementally adding weight to our squats and deadlifts. On that evening, I felt energetic enough to deadlift 500 pounds. The plan was to perform this lift for five sets of five. Although I'd lifted that much before without any adverse effects, I experienced some shortness of breath that evening. But I saw no reason for alarm. We were in a hot gym, working out under glaring lights. I dismissed the shortness of breath as a symptom of dehydration or a side effect of lifting so much weight. I shook off the subtle discomfort and continued working out.

But the feeling persisted once I got home. Perhaps it was indigestion, I reasoned. I took an antacid and prepared for bed, still unfazed by the pain, which now radiated beneath my breastbone. Although I woke several times throughout the night, I still didn't think anything was amiss. I get up two to three times a night to use the bathroom, so I chalked it up to an active bladder.

But as soon as I woke the next morning, I went into survival mode. The pain below my breast had grown more pronounced, and I knew something was wrong. I threw on some jeans, grabbed my keys, and headed to the store to buy more antacids. Anxiety grew within me as I got into my car and drove down the steep hill on which I live. This was the beginning of a series of pivotal decisions that led me to the ER. I had to make a logistical decision as I drove, one that I now realize was a life or death choice. Upon reaching the bottom of the hill, I could have made a right onto Main Street and continued to a local grocery store to pick up antacids. But I didn't make that right turn; instead, I veered left, following an instinct I couldn't explain at the time. I made the left with the intention of going to CVS, which was about a mile away, as opposed to the grocery store, which was a block away in the other direction.

While driving, I called Ray. As a nurse practitioner, Ray was well-versed in what might be causing chest pain and what to do in emergency situations. He told me to immediately go to the emergency room. Despite my brother's advice to go to the ER, I walked into CVS in search of a liquid antacid. By then, the symptoms had escalated. I entered the store hunched over, unable to remain upright. My distress became apparent to others in the store, especially the cashier, who asked if I was okay. I held up my right hand to signal that I was, but I said nothing as I searched for the antacid. I drank it while standing in the aisle, still not realizing how grave my situation was.

As I walked out of CVS, I noticed the urgent care facility across the street. I had gone in two days earlier to meet the owner, who was looking for a partner for his physical therapy practice. Again I was at a crossroads. Should I drive home and rest or go to the clinic? My symptoms seemed to worsen by the minute and I was starting to doubt my self-diagnosed indigestion. I decided to drive across the street. When I exited my car again, I clutched my chest while bent over at the waist. The possibility of imminent death sparked a fear that overwhelmed my discomfort. The clinic secretary immediately recognized the severity of my condition. She called the doctor, the same one I met two days prior, as he hadn't arrived yet. I would be his first patient of the day, and this meeting would be rather different than our initial conversation.

To this day, I marvel at the timing of the escalation of my symptoms. Had they peaked an hour earlier, I might have gone home after stopping into CVS. The urgent care clinic wouldn't have been open yet, and I likely would have died in my home.

But the stars aligned for me that morning. About five minutes after the secretary placed the call, the doctor arrived. He ran an EKG on me, which showed an obvious abnormality in the electrical circuitry of my heart. Seeing the abnormality and my discomfort, he gave me some aspirin. While sitting in triage, I called Ray again and told him what was happening. He immediately went into big brother mode, comforting me and assuring me that he was on his way.

In the meantime, the doctor called an ambulance that arrived about two minutes after he hung up the phone. Lying in the ambulance and speaking with the medic, I was afraid. I thought I was going to die. Upon entering the emergency room, I looked up and there was my brother, hurriedly walking in with an expression of concern. I was relieved at the sight of him. The ER doctor did blood work that showed some abnormalities indicating that there was heart damage. The pain in my chest had become unbearable. I was fading away. As my vision blurred, I recall Ray holding my hand, tears in his eyes. He insisted that the doctor give me something for the pain, but the meds made no difference. The pain returned within ten minutes of them being administered. I was lying there dying, but holding out hope that the doctors surrounding me could turn this around. That's when they told me to make the next pivotal decision: Do I stay at this hospital or go to Columbia Presbyterian? I was very afraid. I thought I was living my last few moments.

Either serendipitously or through divine intervention, Columbia Presbyterian had implemented a new cath lab (a catheterization lab is an examination room where doctors and nurses use diagnostic equipment to visualize arteries of the heart and treat abnormalities) at this local Westchester hospital a month prior. The lab was a satellite of the same lab in which my brother worked in New York City. He knew the staff in the lab that day, who happened to be his colleagues from Manhattan. This made my choice much easier. I was staying local, a decision that hastened my treatment.

The doctors ran more tests and found an obstructed artery. As they prepped me for surgery, the staff comforted me by explaining that they had done the surgery many times and saying I would be fine. I stared at the fluorescent lighting and the ceiling tiles as they spoke. The prep lasted thirty-five minutes but it felt like an eternity. No matter how reassuring the staff tried to be, I knew I was hanging in the balance between life and death.

The doctors cleared my obstruction and placed a stent in the artery. The cardiologist determined that the clog was an aberration because all my other arteries were healthy. There were no signs of cardiac disease, which is atypical of people who tend to have these events.

Several doctors examined me, and they were all in dismay. The one implicating factor upon which they agreed was that my recent personal troubles may have precipitated this near-death experience. Looking back, I'm still shocked that the situation became so extreme. If it weren't for a few seemingly simple decisions that were made, such as driving to CVS instead of shopping closer to home, I would have died. That very thought was almost too surreal to comprehend. I could not fathom leaving behind my kids, my mother, my brother, my entire family. Lying on the verge of death showed me that what truly matters, unequivocally, is family. I felt then that I had been ushered to a crossroads by a divine force, humbling me and bringing me to the realization that there is something much larger than me that's working on my behalf. The fact that I survived helped me realize that my existence has a purpose. I was fortunate that I pulled through, and the experience reaffirmed to me that there is a reason I'm here on this earth. I was chosen to be an emissary for wellness, and I vowed then to extend my rehabilitation practice to include holistic well-being.

Ultimately, I spoke with four cardiologists, none of whom could identify why I had had a heart attack. The only explanation was stress. Needless to say, this was a big eye opener for me. I had been doing everything right (or so I thought), yet stress still overtook my body. Suddenly the connection of mind, body, and spirit became very clear. The picture of perfect health is not only in the physical. It is much more than that.

Now things must change, I told myself. I had to address every part of me for the healthier version of myself to manifest. This transformation would require a mental commitment. I realized that to live out my journey successfully, I would first have to harness mental toughness, resilience, and the courage to continue.

CHAPTER TWO

Embrace the Human Experience

"The human experience consists of ebbs and flows. But with optimal wellness, we obtain the resilience to overcome the hardships that accompany it."

— Dr. Ivan Hernandez

I've always been fascinated with the sciences, particularly psychology. The human mind is vast, and its capacity exceeds what we know. The mind is the driving influence behind all our decision making. In our adult years, many of the events we experienced in childhood and adolescence continue to influence the ways in which we interact with the world. This became apparent to me as I reflected on many of the decisions I had made in my adult life. The most significant of these was the choice to remain married to my ex long after it was clear we were in an unhealthy relationship. For many of our years together, the "writing was on the wall." We were both unhappy, and the strain wore away at me mentally and tore down my self-esteem. But I stayed in the marriage, defying all logic. In a few moments, you will understand what I mean. But for now, I will say this: Love is a mental, psychological commitment that can cause a person to endure unhealthy circumstances despite knowing that doing so goes against his own interests.

My dad left my mother when I was young. I share that not to tell you a sob story, because that unfortunate circumstance afflicts households throughout the world, but to provide context for why I struggled to leave a failing marriage. I do not consider myself a statistic. I am me, a distinct individual. Like everyone else, I experienced things as a child that influenced my psyche. The dissolution of my parents' relationship impacted me deeply, and it inspired me to make a promise to my mother. Seeing the pain she endured when my father left her, I vowed that I would never be the type of person who would cause that kind of heartache. I promised to never leave my wife or children the way he left us. In my eyes, children are a top priority. I don't know what my dad was thinking, nor do I need to explore his potential rationale. But his actions impacted the way I molded myself as a husband and father.

I met my ex when I was seventeen years old. We enjoyed the initial honeymoon phase, as most couples do. But a little more than a year into our courtship, the romance had dissipated and problems that were not obvious to me became apparent to others. By the time we reached our early twenties, friends and family could see the relationship was toxic. They tried to persuade me to get out of it. I denied their observations and resisted their advice because I knew this was my future wife. The relationship wasn't all bad, and the good times made me believe we belonged together. But we had more than our share of arguments, and in retrospect, we should have seen the warning signs. Although most couples argue occasionally, our conflict resolution skills were poor from the beginning and didn't improve once we got married. The toxicity that we tried to ignore from so early on ultimately ended our marriage.

About ten years ago, we reached a point at which being with each other became too difficult. She left me for another man, and we planned to divorce. We went through all the motions, going to court with our lawyers. But for reasons beyond my control, we failed to make our divorce official. The legal fees were mounting, and state laws made the formality of getting a divorce very difficult for both of us. We remained separated because my ex was in a relationship, and I started dating again as well.

I began seeing someone who was special to me at the time, and who on paper made perfect sense for me. We dated for two years, but life complicated our relationship. Although I was still happily separated, my ex reached out to me for help when her family moved out of New York. She had been living with her father and struggled to keep an apartment on her own. We soon reconciled. Within a year and a half, we had our second son.

My children are the highlight of my life, so I do not regret rekindling our relationship. Aside from the joy Henry brought to my life, however, the second round of our relationship wrought even more toxicity and discord than the first. New issues arose on top of those that had never been resolved. I learned that my ex had kept in contact with the same man she had originally left me for, and I realized that she didn't respect me. I told myself I was not good enough for her, as I apparently wasn't the man she wanted. Feelings of inadequacy weighed on me. It is amazing how much someone else can cause you to doubt yourself. You might be the furthest thing from their minds, but their actions still impact your psyche.

On more positive days, I told myself that she didn't know what she had. Friends and family members reassured me that I'm "the complete package" and tried to lift my spirits, but their words brought fleeting comfort. For so long, the only thing that mattered was what my ex thought of me. The painful truth was that she didn't really know who I was. Eventually, I understood that there was more to me than what she made me feel.

But there was the issue of the pact I made to my mother and myself. I had to make a choice. My wife had already left me once and though she was with me again, she was still seeing her previous lover. Coming to grips with the thought of leaving someone you love is draining and all-consuming. You wonder how you can walk away from the person who has been a pivotal force in your life since you were barely more than a child. Ultimately, however, you must choose self-love and self-respect, no matter what promises you made in the past.

I still remember the night I chose to leave her. Her behavior toward me seemed to have changed in recent months, particularly when we were together at my son's basketball games or practices. His coach was the man she had left me for initially, and I soon realized that even though we were together, she had never really left him. One fall evening, I arrived at my son's basketball game to find her already there. I gave her a kiss hello, and she seemed extremely cold to me, though I didn't know why. After the game, my son and I went home and proceeded through our typical evening routines. Though my ex lived with me, she had taken to sleeping in the guest room in recent months as our relationship deteriorated. Despite this distance, however, I could still sense when something was wrong with her. I held onto hope that one day we would work through our problems and be close again.

When she arrived home after the game, I knew her mood was off. My instincts told me to call my son's coach. Uncomfortable though I knew the conversation might be, he knew her well and might offer some insights into what was troubling her. The thought that she might be seeing him again tore me up inside, but I had to know. When I told him who was calling, the coach sounded melancholy and resigned. The conversation went as follows:

Me: "Are you seeing my wife again?"
Coach: "Yes."
Me: "For how long?"
Coach: "The last eight months."

The shock at his frank response rang in my ears, and I stumbled backward, knocking into a loveseat nestled by my window. My gut ached; I felt as though I had taken a punch in the stomach. The world seemed surreal as I sat on the loveseat, trying to process his admission. I had known this was a possibility, but to hear it from him in such plain terms was more than I could stand. My breathing sped up and I was too stunned to speak. After a slight pause, Coach had more to share.

Coach: "That's not it."
Me: "Well, what else is there?"
Coach: "She's pregnant."

I needed to get off the phone. I suggested that we speak in person, and he accepted the invitation. I remember getting into the car and calling my brother, repeating the conversation to him. My brother met me at the local school where I planned to meet Coach. All three of us had attended that school, though in different years. Never had I expected to be back there under these circumstances.

Although I was angry, I had no ill intentions toward Coach. I just wanted answers. When he arrived, he clearly expected the worst. "I know you are here to fuck me up," he said as he got out of his car.

"No, I just want to know if you are telling me the truth," I responded.

Coach explained that my wife had sent him an email with a picture of the sonogram, proving she was pregnant. My brother saw the pain growing in me, and he cut off the conversation. "Let's go. This isn't worth it. This guy isn't worth it," he said. "He's a bum and has done you a favor. You can't see it now, but trust me, he has done you a favor."

Of course, my brother was right. Coach had given me a "get out of jail free card." I finally had the clarity to disconnect myself from the purgatorial void in which I lived. I knew that leaving her meant breaking the pact I had with my mother, but I saw no other option. She was now pregnant with another man's child. It was time to go home and address her with all the questions racing in my mind.

My brother accompanied me back to the house, following me in his car. As soon as I arrived, I started packing. My ex stood in the doorway of our bedroom. She was so smug, her attitude so matter-of-fact and unapologetic. The world felt unreal as I packed my clothes into my brother's car and drove to his home. He and his family took me in and let me sleep on their futon, providing love and solace on that horrific night.

Despite the anguish in my heart, I went to work the next day. That was my testament to moving on, going forward. But I couldn't hide the pain, and I even broke down in front of patients as I tried to cope with this new reality. Every time I thought about her behavior, the pain overtook me. Each memory of her cold demeanor caused me to become flushed with emotion.

Several weeks went by and the Thanksgiving holiday approached. Somewhere in the chaos of the past several weeks, I had agreed to split the holiday with my ex. She would have the boys the first half of the day, and I would take them the second half.

But when I picked up the boys, both were visibly sick with colds. I knew they had been outside watching the Thanksgiving Day parade, and I had also been made aware they were with a mutual friend who was also battling a cold. Given the weather and exposure to another sick person, I decided the boys needed rest more than they needed continued Thanksgiving festivities. I was still staying at Ray's house, which meant I would expose his children to my kids' colds, and I didn't want to put his family through that. He and I determined that it was best for my boys to go home and rest in their own beds. I called my ex and told her the plan, but this simple request ignited into an argument. I remember the look of shock on my brother's face as he heard her rail against us both through the phone. Though she and I both wanted what was best for the kids, our interactions were extremely strained.

My sister-in-law acted as the mediator and brought the kids back to their mom's house. My ex had not shared much about her pregnancy up to that point with anyone on my side of the family, including me. But for some reason, she decided to share with my sister-in-law what she referred to as the great news of her pregnancy. This was a new level of audacity in my opinion, to be celebrating the fact that she was carrying another man's child while she was still married to me. My sister-in-law congratulated her but later questioned me about her actions. Why was she so happy to be pregnant when she was still a married woman, having a baby through an adulterous relationship? I didn't have an answer. My mother-in-law seemed not to understand her daughter's actions either. I spoke to her in hopes she could provide some insight into the situation, but she couldn't. The only thing I knew for sure was that in a few months, a new baby would be here.

If you are wondering how I am so sure the child wasn't mine, I had a vasectomy years before this happened. A rare kidney disease prevented me from securing a life insurance policy. I decided to limit my liability and divide my resources if I were to perish from this disease. Knowing that if I had more children I would have to divide less among more, I had the vasectomy to secure my family's future. This decision was not made unilaterally. On many occasions, I spoke to my ex and expressed my concern for all our futures should I die an early death caused by this rare DNA abnormality. Despite the gravity of that decision, my ex appeared to have little empathy. She did not allay my concerns or encourage me to make a decision that was in the best interests of everyone, the boys and her included. Her distance during this deeply emotional time added to the festering problems between us.

But I went ahead with the procedure anyway. The silver lining was that it motivated me to become a vocal proponent of the idea that health equals wealth. My health was my life insurance policy. It was incumbent upon me to limit my exposure to disease and death by changing my lifestyle. If I lived, I would stand a chance to accumulate enough wealth to care for my children and provide for them on their journeys toward independence and adulthood — college, homes, and weddings.

The boys have always been, and continue to be, my motivation to overcome adversity. But their mother had become their antithesis and my anathema. A court mediator suggested that we see a co-parenting mediator as we worked through our separation. But my ex antagonized me during these sessions. On one occasion, I recall her giving me the middle finger and saying things like "You're going to be paying for me the rest of your life." When we left the room, I would intentionally avoid her and take a separate elevator. Even though I made every effort to stay away from her, she filed an order of protection against me based on sheer fabrications. But this was nothing new. She had spit on me and thrown things at me, and when I responded in any way, even shielding myself, she'd call the police. I never laid a finger on her, but she knew they would always favor her story. In an effort to protect myself, I would video record her rampages, because otherwise it was her word against mine.

The tension escalated after one mediation session in particular. She claimed that as we left court, I threatened to kill her and her baby by running her over. The story, of course, was a complete fabrication she tried to use to gain leverage and hurt me during these proceedings. She was the aggressor, the one who chose to leave me once before, who chose to cheat, and who became pregnant with another man's child. Yet here she was accusing me of threatening to hurt her. The order of protection she filed against me included that I could not see my kids, even in the morning at their school. Still, I thought I could hold on and that I had it together. I would fight to see my children, and I would not let her beat me down. But only a few days after the order of protection was issued, I suffered the heart attack.

Afterword on Relationships

I learned a great deal about relationships from the years spent with my ex. Each partner serves as a pillar supporting the relationship. When one of the people in the relationship fails to hold up his or her pillar, the relationship crumbles. Both partners need to make an effort to support the pillars and keep the relationship healthy.

People do not remain the same, and as we get older, we begin to see changes in each other. Our ideologies and thought processes mature, especially as we become more well-rounded and well-traveled. There used to be TV shows that tested how well people knew their partners, and I remember that the details were important. Do you know their favorite color or ice cream? Are you willing to make a change with them? That question in particular is so important, because I believe wholeheartedly in the concept that the only constant is change. Love, respect, and a willingness to evolve as partners keep the pillars standing. There has to be a willingness to succeed and to heed the big picture.

Relationships should not be lived as a tug of war in which every battle is fought to be won. Conflicts are inevitable in all relationships, whether they be between a mother and daughter, a father and son, or a teacher and student. But mutual love and respect will bring the conflicts to a close. When no one is willing to compromise, people can go years without talking to loved ones. We miss out on so much because we refuse to compromise on the small things.

Being faithful, financial issues, and changing priorities can strengthen partnerships or lead to the dissolution of marriages, depending how they're approached. However, the ability to talk to each other and develop strategic conflict resolution skills allows people to navigate these areas and get to better places with their loved ones. Relationships that survive adversity will flourish. The growth and strength are unimaginable when this happens.

CHAPTER THREE

Recognize the Signs of Abusive Relationships

"Abuse can strike even the most unsuspecting of individuals."

— Dr. Ivan Hernandez

I had an encounter recently in which a friend shared that she was in an abusive relationship. Although she confided in me, she never reported the abuser, her child's father, to the police. She wanted him to keep a clean record so he could get a job. Her partner had been out of work for the majority of their relationship, and he was a classic abuser. He laid hands on her several times, pulling her hair and hurting her in other ways. The abuse also included verbal attacks, and my friend was terrified of him. Once, she grabbed a knife to defend herself, and he called the cops. She spent the night in jail. After years of compromising her safety to protect his record, she was the one in jail. He didn't think twice about what going to jail would cost her, even though drawing the knife had been an act of desperation.

I think I surprised her with my response. Once she had finished telling me about the horrors of their relationship, I told her to thank God. If he hadn't called the cops on her, she might have spent another ten years in that dangerous situation. "Would you rather have endured a lifetime of misery or spent one night in jail to open your eyes to the truth?" I asked. Similar to my circumstances, my friend needed a drastic wake-up call. For her, it was the father of her child calling the police when she tried to fend off his blows. For me, it took my wife becoming pregnant with another man's baby to accept that the dream I had for my life could not be.

My friend's story of being abused resonated with me. I'm a decent-sized guy, so people might find it odd when I say that my ex abused me. But I often had to protect myself against slaps in the face and objects she flung in my direction. Having an audience didn't deter her attacks. Sometimes she would hit me in front of her mother until her mother told her to stop. But the silver lining was that our volatile and dysfunctional relationship taught me to believe in something greater. When I finally realized that I needed to leave my ex and began to process the harm she had caused me, I learned that relationships do not have to be painful. That experience helped me appreciate the value of a good woman.

Contrary to what many believe, men can suffer from abuse at the hands of their female partners. People often become so accustomed to deviant behavior that they don't see the toxicity in their lives until something world-shattering happens. That's when we reach our tipping points. Many victims don't realize the extent of the danger until someone lands in jail or worse. Sometimes we must go to extremes before we are willing to question our circumstances. After years of anger and violence, my ex's behavior seemed normal to me. She would spit on me and throw whatever household items were handy, and in time, I thought nothing of this.

People also reach their tipping points when they learn their partners are habitual cheaters and are having someone else's baby. Some even accept the cheating, but they can't cope with the child. My story of being cheated on is not unique. Many people have found themselves in the same place I was — hurt, shocked, disbelieving. But we all reach our tipping point sometime, even if it causes a catastrophe. A battered woman will eventually fight back, and that is the moment when she realizes she is being abused. She and her attacker experience a moment of clarity when they see what they have become. When only one party is committing abuse and there are no repercussions, that person fails to see his or her actions as abuse. People can justify anything if they're ruled by emotional whims, ignorant of the potential for regret and permanent damage. This is how people abuse others for days, months, and years at a time. Denial is powerful. It's what enables abusers tell themselves they're not abusers and victims to tell themselves the same lies. Now that I'm removed from my own abusive experience, I see this clearly.

Relationships are not easy. They require ongoing commitments from both parties to adapt and evolve. More importantly, there needs to be respect and love for one another, the type of love that protects and does not harm. Love must evolve but keep those key requirements. We cannot become angry when our partners change, nor can we force them to be who they once were. Both people must grow and change together, becoming more ambitious and pushing one another out of their comfort zones. If someone moves in a harmful direction, that's a problem. But growth is good, and we cannot stay on the ground while our partners fly, and vice versa. We cannot become bitter when our loved ones achieve simply because we want things to remain the same. That's when blame begins and we find reasons to mistreat each other.

Resentment takes a toll, whether voiced or unspoken. It's the cause of the thick air that hangs over the dinner table. It becomes the elephant in the room and the source of contention within the home. Once it is present, a cold war begins, a subtle, gradual end. You recoil from holding hands, stop kissing each other. There are no displays of affection or acts of generosity inspired by love of your partner. All help given at this point is done so grudgingly, out of obligation. Then you begin keeping score. Eventually lovers become foes who sleep in separate bedrooms.

You must be alert when these cold wars begin. If you seek acknowledgement and recognition outside the relationship, stop. Return to your lover and tell him or her what you need. Talk things out before resentment begins. Don't project assumptions onto your partner and start arguments over trivial issues. That is the mistake many of us make. We expect the other person to read between the lines and figure out what is wrong. Instead, we must speak openly about our wants and feelings. Time does not stop for our petty arguments. How many years will we stew in anger and close ourselves off to real, healthy love?

Of course, you must love yourself before you can have a deep connection with someone else. If you love and respect yourself, you will recognize that you deserve happiness and to be treated well. People settle when we assume we can do no better. Healthy people — physically, mentally healthy people — challenge themselves daily so they can do better. Settling is never an option for them.

Takeaways: The Signs of Abuse

Lack of respect:

If your partner is openly cheating or berates you in front of other people, he or she does not respect you.

Lack of effort:

Accusations that "He's not trying" or "She's not trying" are strong statements. Before making decisions about the relationship, be honest about whether your partner is making an effort, even if it's not in the way you'd like. Are the efforts emotional or monetary? Are they sincere? If the other person is taking initiative to save the relationship, there is hope. But if he or she is disengaged or neglectful, there is little reason for hope.

Lack of love:

Love transcends hardships and rough patches. It inspires us to get back to where we want to be. When the love wanes, all things fall apart. Fear and distrust set in where the love used to be, and jealous, wounded lovers can turn abusive. Love is not harmful or disrespectful or abusive; it should be the best thing that ever happened to you. When the love goes away on either or both sides, that's when you experience suffering.

Afterword on Abuse

The warning signs flared early in my relationship with my ex. Her mother telling her to stop putting her hands on me, her striking me in front of my friends — these were abusive actions, and they indicated the problems to come. So why did I stay so long? I grew up thinking there would be a happy ending, that there is a happily ever after in every relationship. It took a while for me to figure out that happily ever after doesn't always exist, at least not in the ways we expect. Rather than waiting for a happy someday, we should take every moment and analyze it for what it is.

We are products of our environments, and I grew up in a household without a father. Out of respect for my mother, I promised to never leave my own family. Despite my ex's abusive behavior, I stayed because I didn't want my children to go through what I did. However, the hitting and the lack of effort on her part should have told me it was only a matter of time before our relationship would fail. My children were the blessings that came out of the turmoil.

My ex seemed incapable of controlling her emotions. We went to counseling, but she rejected the counselors' attempts to help because she believed they were not on her side. They often told her she wasn't facing reality. I agreed.

But instead of insisting upon love and respect, I accepted her bad behavior. Time and again, I forgave her, always believing better days were ahead. They weren't. Friends and family told me to get out, but I didn't listen. I understand now what they saw back then, but I couldn't appreciate their concerns until I loved myself enough to leave her. I was warped by my parents' divorce, so I normalized her behavior and allowed it to continue.

I always hoped that we'd reach a turning point for the better. But now I know both partners must respect each other for a relationship to work. Even with all the effort I put into the relationship, I sometimes wonder if she ever respected me. I know now that people project their inadequacies on you when they believe can. Verbal and physical abuse is a way of doing that.

Counseling works best when it is done prophylactically, not after the fact. I should have left the first time I learned my ex cheated on me, when we were in our twenties. She seemed to show no remorse then, and the pattern continued in the years that followed, even though I expected better from her.

I made a mistake by choosing not to listen to my friends and family. I know now that we must love with our hearts and be guided by our brains. The heart is the vehicle by which movement occurs, but the brain steers us in the right direction. When you lose objectivity and do not listen to your brain, you base decisions on emotional perceptions and elements you cannot control. You look so hard for your desired outcome that you miss the truth.

There's a common belief that some people will never change. They think they are fine the way they are, or they don't have the desire to be better. The transformative process is within anyone's grasp, but it requires effort. Change means pushing through resistance, because the path of least resistance yields nothing meaningful. My ex grew up among people who were unwilling to change, and she possessed a self-image that didn't allow for doubt. She is a product of her environment, and her reluctance to bend for our relationship resulted in the abusive behaviors that drove us apart. We are the sum of our experiences.

Schools don't teach you about relationships, which seems odd to me now. If ever a part of your life could set you off course, this is it. Without deep understandings of what healthy, supportive relationships look like, people end up in co-dependent and harmful situations. To truly love someone and know whether you are compatible, you must be able to communicate about your backgrounds. Where and whom did they come from? What behaviors did they learn from their upbringings? How do they handle conflicts? We should apply the same level of due diligence on finding a mate as we do on choosing the right college, car, or home.

Relationships work best between people of similar backgrounds and values. With familiarity grows fondness. I am not a proponent of opposites attract — the volatility that erupts from these couplings often results in conflict and even abusiveness. There needs to be some common ground to sustain the relationship that both spouses share, because otherwise children will be the only commonality, and when they're grown, there's nothing left.

CHAPTER FOUR

Learn to Cope With
the Unexpected

*"There's always a silver lining in every
cloud. My failures in business gave me
the business degree I never planned for."*
— Dr. Ivan Hernandez

I see every life experience as part of the journey, rather than destinations, we must reach.
The resistance we encounter along the way,
both our own and that of others, is necessary
because by challenging us, it forces us to grow.
If we embrace the challenges, we flourish.
Without obstacles, we become complacent,
conceding to the difficulties instead of fighting for something better. Life wasn't meant to
be easy. What would be the point of goals and
where would we find satisfaction in achievement if it weren't for the struggles?

In 2009, after successfully launching my first
outpatient orthopedic physical therapy office in
Yonkers, I decided to open a branch seven miles
north, in Elmsford, New York. I had passed the

spot that became the new location every morning on my commute to New York Medical College, where I served as an adjunct faculty member. The corner was always heavily congested, yet there the sign always hung: "Available for rent." That year was already a full one, even without expanding my business. My youngest son became a toddler, and my family and I were still settling into the house we had purchased the year prior. But I didn't want to let myself get complacent. Increasing my business ventures would motivate me to work harder and reach my full potential as both a physician and a father.

I signed the lease on the new location, full of optimism about how well we might do in this new area. Several therapists worked for me at the time, and I divided my schedule between the two branches so I could oversee both operations. Within a few short months, the Elmsford office picked up pace while the Yonkers office maintained its status quo. Although the problems with my ex persisted, I was happy.

But challenges cropped up during the next several years. As most business owners know, the key to keeping the lights on is maintaining a good staff. As the Elmsford office entered its third year, I began having trouble in that regard, for several reasons. Legal hurdles arose when I tried to file for sponsorship status on behalf of the foreign-born physical therapists I wanted to hire. The company also faced recruiting difficulties. My position as an adjunct at New York Medical College provided a pipeline to talented graduates, but I preferred to hire more experienced candidates, given our heavy case-loads. Teaching offered me a way to break up the monotony of my everyday routine, and it enabled me to build a network of potential colleagues once students had gained more experience. I also enjoyed the opportunity to serve as a reference and resource to students. But my role at the college didn't lead to immediate hiring opportunities, and I found maintaining a full, thriving staff increasingly difficult. Some prospective hires failed their licensing exams; others did not receive sponsorship; and some employees got married and moved out of the area. I was responsible for making the decisions and figuring out a way forward, and eventually the stress took a toll.

But I managed. Eventually, I got the hang of hiring well, and an ambitious, reliable therapist from India joined my team. This therapist, who I'll call Tee, carved out a niche for herself in women's health, seeing patients who had pelvic floor issues. My expertise is as an orthopedic sports clinician, so her niche was far from my own, which was great for attracting new clients to the business. She became my lead therapist at the Elmsford clinic, and the practice thrived.

Tee developed a strong following, and she was great at what she did. But all good things come to an end. Her boyfriend, who had been living in Seattle, proposed in 2013, and the couple had a tough decision to make about where they would live after they got married. She loved her work and had blossomed in this particular niche. But her fiancé had a good job working for Amazon. He submitted a request to transfer to the company's New York branch but was told he would have to wait for the relocation. He and Tee agreed that he would try to find work in New York within six months; if he didn't, they would discuss her moving to Seattle. As the months passed, I became increasingly anxious about what was going to happen.

Tee was among the several therapists who had become the backbone of Executive Park Physical Therapy. It was because of her that I was able to manage my personal life while growing the business. Losing her would be a real blow.

Her husband's transfer never came through. After their agreed-upon six-month window closed, she resigned. Though I was sad to lose her, I tried to focus on what came next. Insurance reimbursement rates were changing, and I was concerned about our abilities to manage outpatient service. I needed to insulate the business against dramatic changes, so I decided to open a third practice, this one in Briarcliff, New York. I rented a small space in a gym that sat across the street from another physical therapy facility. The area was affluent, and there were several physical therapy offices. But my approach was different from theirs and from what I offered at my other locations. I would see one patient an hour and only take specific insurance plans. Over the course of a few months, that facility flourished beyond what I could have ever imagined. Word of mouth spread about the high level of care I delivered, and clients poured in. But as the reality of losing Tee drew closer, I had a decision to make. Did I spend less time on the lucrative new practice in Briarcliff to maintain the business at Elmsford? The Elmsford clinic was thriving because of Tee's pelvic floor services, a niche offering I couldn't replicate. I also knew it would be tough to replace her. Pelvic floor therapists are difficult to recruit because they usually have their own practices. But I had to at least entertain the possibility, because I was locked into a ten-year lease with a personal guarantee at the Elmsford location. No such contract existed for Briarcliff.

I attempted to negotiate with the Elmsford landlord after Tee left, hoping to shift focus to the opportunities in Briarcliff. But the landlord had a negative reputation, and I soon discovered that it was well-deserved. I thought that after five years of being a good tenant, he would be sympathetic to my situation. I offered exit strategies and settlements, and he refused them all. I finally decided to let the space go, knowing that he would fight me. Lo and behold, he filed a lawsuit against me and my LLC.

The personal guarantee on the loan meant that he could come after every asset I had. I was worried about my family, our house, and the other businesses. By early 2014, I began assembling a dream team to protect my family and me. I hired business attorneys who advised me to file Chapter 7 bankruptcy personally and Chapter 11 for the LLC as a means of reorganizing the business. I also hired an accountant and his assistant, both of whom became instrumental in saving the business. To this day, I feel indebted to the four professionals I brought on during this time. My business manager, who I originally hired as a bookkeeper, was also invaluable as we made arrangements and put the documentation in order.

I was paying massive legal fees to stay afloat, but there was no other choice. Without these people, I could have lost everything. I was not going to let that happen to myself or my family.

Yet things at home had deteriorated. Although I was consumed by the lawsuit, I did not fail to notice that my wife had grown increasingly distant and had moved out of our bedroom. Still, I believed we would make things right after the lawsuit was settled. I filed for Chapter 11 in August 2014. Three months later, I learned that she had been cheating on me for the past eight months and was pregnant by our son's basketball coach, a man with whom she had cheated on me in the past.

The Chapter 11 procedures were frustrating and messy. The landlord was contentious and fought me at every turn along the way. But the case closed eventually, and my family's assets were saved. But the stress of the business concerns and my troubled home life took their toll, which became all too apparent as I lay in the hospital, fearing for my life.

Takeaways on Coping with Adversity

Find balance.

The domains of mind, body, and spirit are responsible for our wellness, and they're overlapping and interdependent. If one fails, the other two will suffer. Therefore, all three must be in balance to maintain a harmonious state. The mind is an especially powerful domain, and thoughts affect our physiologies. Negative thoughts will negatively impact your body, and positive thoughts allow good hormones to be released. Thinking the right way is critical to your health. Thoughts become words, and words become behaviors. This is why I believe it is important to give yourself daily positive affirmations. Try repeating phrases such as:

"Yes I can."

"I'm happy to be alive today."

"I'm grateful to have another opportunity to better myself."

Simple mantras like these can generate overall well-being just by thinking them or saying them out loud.

I lacked this insight earlier in my life. I didn't fully comprehend the interconnectedness of the mind, body, and spirit. As I get older, I realize balance is key to making the most of this wonderful human experience. Often when we engage in something unfamiliar, we experience heightened stress levels. Our bodies create cortisol and epinephrine, the stress hormones. As you persevere and stay on course, you move from the struggle phase to a release phase. In the release phase, your body moves from a state of elevated consciousness to sub-consciousness and your body will adapt. That is the dynamic nature of the human body.

As we remain resilient in our own evolutions, our bodies start to familiarize themselves with the new normal. We become fully engrossed in our well-being. The flow state is when the body starts secreting "feel good" chemicals like dopamine, an addictive chemical that can be triggered by habits such as gambling, excessive sex, chocolate, drugs, eating, or alcohol. You can get the same effect and the same amount of dopamine release in a wellness transformation. As long as you stay the course, your body will start to secrete dopamine, and you will enter the flow state of mind — otherwise known as "being in the zone." That's when you begin to enjoy all the aspects of wellness.

Develop wellness rituals.

Once you're in the wellness mindset, eating healthy and working out become rituals. You don't leave your house without brushing your teeth in the morning because that's part of your oral hygiene ritual. Think of the whole body in the same light. When you get into a wellness flow, you become wired to pursue your own well-being and optimal health.

I tell my patients and clients who seek a life of wellness that the mind is everything. Your mindset affects the entire journey, and it's easy to veer off course. Results are often dependent on the ability to remain positive by training your thoughts and using daily affirmations.

There is such a thing as good stress, and the hormone cortisol, which is produced under stress, protects us when we're in danger. Cortisol triggers our fight or flight response and heightens our sense of awareness. But too much cortisol can be toxic. This is why meditation, deep breathing practices, and stress management are so important. When you begin to take on more than you can handle, you elevate these levels, and it becomes difficult to remain focused. But you can reclaim your power through positive thinking.

Pay no attention to naysayers.

Wellness is a cornerstone of a life well-lived. When you are well, you become more present and successful as a father, son, daughter, husband, wife, breadwinner, or whatever roles you fulfill. Unfortunately, we live in a society that does not prioritize health and wellness. Most Americans are overweight according to the Centers for Disease Control and Prevention. Those who are healthy and concerned with their physical fitness are often judged as being vain. For example, the Obamas practice a healthy lifestyle and some view them as elitist. People who cast judgments against those who live well and prioritize their health are distractions from what matters. If being healthy is vain, we can all stand a little more vanity in our lives. There's nothing wrong with feeling good about yourself when your clothes start to fit better; that means you're decreasing your risk for preventable diseases. Beer bellies are highly correlated with avoidable ailments, so pay no attention when someone teases you for working on your six-pack. A flat stomach represents a healthy lifestyle, not just vanity. Instead of viewing fitness as frivolous, think of it as a step toward avoiding diabetes.

The better we feel physically, the more positively we feel mentally and emotionally. Our mental and emotional states dictate whether we are stressed and in pain, and unchecked stress leads to physical problems, including life-threatening ones. Quality of life deteriorates when we don't pay attention to all aspects of our well-being. But we can change course if we are mindful of what matters most.

CHAPTER FIVE

You Don't Need Religion to be Spiritual

"The human mind is very much like a compass because it navigates the human vessel to move and when one's mental state is found it moves in the right direction."

— Dr. Ivan Hernandez

I have come to the realization that optimal wellness is the sum of multiple dimensions all working harmoniously. I have also come to understand that spirituality is not synonymous with being religious.

Religion serves an important purpose in many people's lives, and that can be a beautiful thing. But spirituality is something different. I put spirituality ahead of everything else I do on a day-to-day basis. My sense of spirituality keeps me in flow regardless of what challenges I face. It reminds to be thoughtful about what kind of imprint I am going to leave on this earth. Spirituality is the energy that resonates within us and connects us to the rest of the world.

Each morning, I ask myself: How am I going to impact the world? What will I do? Although I consider myself many things, I am first and foremost a father who wants to give all that he can to his children. That is my highest purpose in life. I want my boys to live an even richer experience than I have, understanding that they, too, will face challenges along the way. I also see myself as a healthcare provider, which is why I have embarked on a campaign to help people through my message that "health is wealth." My third role is to be the best person I can be in my relationships. If I am giving my all to others, whether that be my mother, my future wife, or my brother, they will give their all back to me.

I am a proponent of the law of reciprocity: when you give out positive energy, people will return it to you and pass it on to others. That is what I hope to do, and that is how I see myself in this world. My energy resonates through every channel and every experience that I have.

I wasn't always in this headspace. As I struggled to cope with Tee's departure, changes within the business, the lawsuit, and the collapse of my marriage, some days it was all I could do to keep my head above water. But having a heart attack changed everything. Not only did it drive home how interconnected my emotional and mental states are with my physical health, it inspired in me a sense of urgency to live well and serve my sons, my patients and clients, and all those who care about me. As I lie in the hospital recovering from surgery, it became clearer than ever that I had neglected deep parts of myself while I struggled to hold it all together. Things had to change. I needed to live my life more purposefully and more fully.

A spiritual purpose puts our lives into context. Sometimes we lose that sense of purpose, and we must stumble into dark places to find the light that shines within ourselves. Adversity provides a way for us to gain an appreciation of what light is. Even the seeds of beautiful flowers begin their lives in dark soil; they must push through the darkness to burst forth into the light. We too can emerge from dark places to see the light and appreciate all that life has to offer.

I believe that everything, good or bad, is meant to be. Even if you don't subscribe to that idea, you might agree that no crisis should go to waste. You could say there is a silver lining in every cloud. However you frame it, we can all appreciate that sometimes we need the dark to fully experience the light. I have known loved ones who turned their lives around after sinking to their lowest depths. They emerged from those trials as though they were touched by a divine entity. My spiritual wellness revolves around the promise in such experiences and in our abilities to become stronger from surviving devastation.

Of course, it's easy to put troubles in context when life is going well. It's when life becomes challenging that we need to remember our higher purpose. That's when we have to assess our character and determine who we are even when the odds seem stacked against us. These are the thoughts that filled my mind in the weeks following my heart attack and surgery. How would I respond to this curveball?

What we give off to the world is a reflection of what is inside of us, and what is inside of us is the sum of our experiences and the extent to which we've processed them.

The good news is that if you are good to people when things are going well, they will reciprocate, especially when you need them most. As the pieces of your life fall into place

once again, though perhaps in different con-
figurations than they were before, these truths
will become apparent. The goodwill you created will come back to you, and a path out of
the darkness will appear.

I emerged from my marriage and the trials
within my business stronger — not unscathed,
but stronger. Ultimately, I am thankful for the
lessons I learned. If things had not happened
the way they did, I would not be where I am
today. We must embrace adversity and see it
through to live life to the fullest extent. Difficulties reveal strengths we didn't know we had.

Takeaways on Spirituality

Create a spiritual mindset for your family.

I talk a lot about building one's own spirituality. However, your spiritual life should extend
to those you love. In my case, it is my children
who are most impacted by spirituality. They
are the recipients of its gifts. How I choose to
raise them and react to their needs, as well as
how I behave in front of them, informs their
ideas of who I am. If I want to instill in them
the virtues of humility, health, and empathy, I
have to embody those attributes myself.

My spiritual grounding reminds me to put out into the world that which I want to get back. The more fully I have embraced my spirituality and conscious living, the more positive the effect I have on my boys and the stronger our relationship. Children take in more than we realize, and our behaviors impact them deeply. What we might see as a simple bad mood, they take to heart, and they may withdraw because of it. I've become acutely aware of the effect my attitude has on my sons as I've watched them cope with the divorce and my heart attack.

Actions speak loudest when teaching mindfulness and spirituality.

Everyone encounters adversity in life. What matters is the mindset we use to overcome it. That's why I want to give my sons the knowledge and tools to survive anything that comes their way. I want them to know that struggles are how we learn. Life is full of peaks and valleys, and with perseverance and faith we are able to overcome all that tests us. Through these trials, we become our best.

I teach my children this concept through my own actions. We can lecture them as much as we want, but kids watch what we do. They rarely remember what we say. How I act will resonate more with them than all the lessons I try to impart through words. I don't try to hide the fact that life is bruising. There will be transitions, trouble, and stress, and their bodies will respond in different ways. I want to teach them how to react, how to take control of their situations and protect their bodies even during times of extreme duress.

Many people fall apart at the first signs of stress because no one ever taught them how to manage it. The way the body reacts physically and emotionally must be mastered the same way you master any other skill. Although trial and error can be great teachers, there are some truths we do not need to experience in order to gain their benefits. Learning to drive a car through trial and error could cost your life or someone else's. Theoretical knowledge enables you to think through your actions and respond appropriately your first time on the road. Stress management is the same way. As a parent, I am responsible for teaching my kids how to manage stress. Knowing how to breathe through tension and practice healthy habits could save their lives.

Embrace spiritual awakenings no matter how they present themselves.

Spiritual awakenings occur in different ways for all of us, but there are some universal experiences associated with these epiphanies. They bring a sense of direction and an end to our loneliness. We suddenly feel connected to something larger than ourselves and understand that there are forces beyond our knowing at work. We catch fleeting glimpses of the big picture and find humility in those moments.

But these wondrous moments can only happen if we give in to the spiritual awakenings that stir within us and do not resist these transformative shifts. The more we give in to the journey, the more profound and lasting the effects. We undergo a continuous process of ego deflation but we also become more conscious of our shifting perspectives. Our view of the world expands to a point at which we no longer possess an exaggerated sense of our existence. Through our awareness, we no longer feel isolated from the rest of the human race, even though we may not understand why the world is the way it is or why we treat one another so terribly. We understand suffering, and we do our best to alleviate it. When our individual contributions combine with those of other spiritually aware people, we become an essential part of the grand design. We are connected at last. I am but one person and I humbly accept my place in the big picture.

CHAPTER SIX

Know That Your Mind Is Your Catalyst

"Change in any direction in one's life is an active and evolving process that requires meticulous attention to our thoughts, which are governed by the past and the goals we have laid down in our minds."

— Dr. Ivan Hernandez

As I recovered from my heart attack, I needed to take back control of my life. But I also had to accept my inability to control the future. I could make certain decisions about how to live and think about the world, but I had to release my need to prevent bad things from happening. I learned that no matter how consuming your difficulties seem at any given time, you can't win a war in one day. You have to focus on segments of the problem, go a mile deep and an inch wide. When you become obsessed with the final outcome, that's when life feels overwhelming. However, if you can compartmentalize your problems and separate the struggles from what's going right, you can make progress. The small wins eventually start to make dents in the larger problems. This isn't always easy. Sometimes you have to have blind faith that everything will be okay.

You have to ask yourself what the "worst case scenario" may be. If it's not going to kill you, then you can begin your plan of attack. During my trials, I tried to get through one day, one battle, at a time. Looking at them collectively seemed completely overwhelming.

It's important to surround yourself with positive people, in good times and in bad. When life gets rough, it's very easy to fall into a rut. Positive people will lift you out of that place through their upbeat, inspiring attitudes. But those who take a negative view of the world will only prolong your stagnation and pain.

Positive thinking also impacts your brain chemistry and enables you to tackle problems from an objective, action-oriented point of view. When we become too emotional, we lose objectivity and act on our whims. We must learn to step back and breathe, and concentrate on the bare essentials that will allow us to maintain an optimal homeostasis. Without that, the body

becomes sickly, and we find ourselves susceptible to a cascade of negative effects. Tackle your
issues one at a time, and eventually you will
conquer them all.

Breathing and meditation are lifesavers for
me during times of difficulty. I find that reading inspirational quotes helps as well. My office
manager, Cecilia, is very calm, and she centers
me and keeps me objective. Any time I start
to fixate on worst-case scenarios, she grounds
me in the present moment and reminds me to
breathe. She helps me evaluate whether my fears
are warranted, and I find perspective through
our talks. Most importantly, she guides me back
to what matters—the life I am building for
myself and my sons, the holistic message I share
with my community, and the spiritual life that
allows me to thrive. We all seek instant gratifica-
tion in our pursuits, but I know that the rewards
I am seeking won't come overnight. With practice, however, I will achieve all that I hope to
do. Harping on things outside my control only
distracts from my purpose.

The biggest change since my heart attack has
been my perspective on life. Now I know why
people say life is short. I was inches from death
on May 28, 2014. I could have died without
having seen my children again, my boys who

mean the world to me. The heart attack was a rude but necessary awakening. Now I strive to live each day like it is my last, to apply a work ethic of which I can be proud, and to possess a mindset that embraces the positive and wastes no time on negativity and trivialities. I appreciate the days more. I have no regrets because I reach out to the people I need and love. I also cut back on work when necessary, because it isn't worth my health to overwhelm myself with one or two additional patients. I enjoy a vacation from time to time, as I believe everyone should.

Whether you go on an exotic vacation or simply take a few days off, you need to relax and connect with your life outside work. Even if you don't have much in the way of resources, take a moment to appreciate life a bit more. Enjoy some downtime alone or with family. Stop and acknowledge what you have achieved. If you can travel, be aware of how much being in another space opens up your life. A few moments spent in nature reminds us that we are just a minuscule part of this universe.

Afterword on regrets

Earlier in this chapter, I said I have no regrets. That's true now, as I've begun to live in a way that doesn't allow for the fear and excuses that so often lead to regrets. But I do hold one regret from the past, and that is not facing the monster within me sooner. Stress and negativity had risen in me until they almost consumed my life. That's why I implore anyone grappling with challenges in life to face your monster. You have to deal with the underlying issues that plague your psyche. Your adversaries only become stronger when they are given the power to control your emotions and your happiness. Freedom comes from taking on the monsters, whatever they may be.

Confronting my business's troubles and my ex's infidelity felt like walking into a war. But I had to deal with them. Problems don't go away when you ignore them; they get worse. Years of fear and ugliness in my marriage led to our divorce, but I did not want to see how dire the situation had become. It wasn't until we hit rock bottom as partners that I finally acknowledged the truth. Now that I have faced my fears, I am the happiest I've ever been. I can live fully and take in everything that this world has to offer. There are so many good people and great things to enjoy, and I am glad I won't miss out on any of it. Once I realized what was missing in my life, I was able to go out and find it. I appreciate life more because I am aware that at any point, death might be imminent. I don't want to look back and wish that I achieved happiness sooner, so now I take the ride where it goes. You have the freedom to choose when and how you take on your monsters. Use that gift wisely.

CHAPTER SEVEN

Take Control of Your Health

"Unweight yourself of your past, and ascend from the depths of your struggle while taking back control of your health."

— Dr. Ivan Hernandez

The human body is both magnificent and highly adaptive. We can transform our bodies into what we want, within the boundaries of our genetic pre-dispositions. But to harness the possibilities, you must have the mental toughness to endure not only bringing your body to an optimal level on a regular basis, but also doing it when you are not in the mood to work out or cook a healthy meal. The test of how badly you want something is whether you persevere when you're tired and have no energy, or when your mind begins to negotiate the benefits of skipping a workout. Your decisions are the test of mental endurance.

Remember that our systems are interdependent. When we strength train or exercise, our bodies create many different chemicals that influence how we feel, both physically and mentally. We feel happier when the endorphins flow, and we sleep better when dopamine production is optimized. Serotonin modulation is another unique benefit of exercise. Physical fitness provides your body with the essentials to move toward wellness.

What Is It About Exercise?

Exercise is a well-known and highly effective antidepressant. I suffered from an acute bout of depression when the world came crashing down on me. However, I was able to capitalize on my knowledge as a physician, and I applied the fundamental principles of exercise to improve my life. When the intensity of the exercise is high, the body secretes chemicals that make a person feel good. I used exercise as a means of enhancing my body, knowing that it would rehabilitate my mind simultaneously.

Healthy means different things for different people. Not everyone will benefit from the same workout regimen. The way I determine the health of an individual is by looking at their blood profiles tests and energy levels as measures of well-being. But there are many ways people can achieve optimal health profiles. Some do it through yoga, Pilates, and good nutrition. I prefer resistance training because this form of exercise stimulates hormone production and elevates the metabolism, possibly for up to forty-eight hours. Resistance exercises activate hormones responsible for your resting metabolic rate, so your body is burning calories while at rest. This is important because most Americans are sedentary for arguably ten hours per day. A person who runs on a treadmill might burn 500 calories in the same amount of time someone doing resistance training burns only 200. But the person doing resistance training will continue to burn calories throughout the day due to the increased the metabolic rate.

Research shows that 1.9 billion people throughout the world are considered overweight. In the U.S., 70 percent of adults fall into this category. Obesity is a pandemic, and increasing metabolic rate through resistance training is one way to combat it.

Resistance Training as a Lifestyle

Resistance training is very efficient. People are busy with work, school, children, and other responsibilities. We spend our lives juggling multiple priorities, and we don't always have time for lengthy workouts. Resistance training is energizing. A thirty- to forty-five-minute workout empowers you to get more done throughout the rest of the day. You'll also see results quickly, which inspires you to stick with the program.

How does resistance training work? Through compound movements. These are exercises that require multiple muscle groups to work at the same time. Squats and deadlifts in particular are known for being effective because they involve so many muscles. As a result, these movements are great for stimulating hormones and therefore metabolic rate. Compound movements are efficient ways to improve physical fitness without making your whole life revolve around the gym. But if you adapt a resistance training regimen, be aware that more is not necessarily better in this scenario. Exercising for too long elevates cortisol levels, which can break down muscle and lower your metabolism. The more muscle we have, the faster our metabolism, and also the more insulin sensitivity we will have. Muscles are the biggest endocrine organs in our body. The endocrine system controls the hormones that are secreted throughout our organs. There are so many chemicals at play in our biological systems, especially when we are looking to lose weight, gain muscle and optimize our well-being. While there are a vast array of hormones to pay attention to, two key hormones are cortisol and insulin. Insulin sensitivity is a critical piece to consider when we are looking to lose weight. Chronically elevated insulin will lead to fat storage and consequently dip our endogenous testosterone production. These changes result in decreased muscle, increased fat and an overall unhealthy spectrum of blood markers. Arguably, insulin resistance is the root derivative linked with every preventable disease that afflicts us like diabetes, cancer, stroke, and Alzheimer's just to name a few, as it is associated with Metabolic Syndrome (the precursor for all of the aforementioned diseases). This is why maintaining muscle strength and muscle mass are important as these adaptations help to regulate the amount of insulin in our blood. The more muscle we have, the more insulin uptake we have. Compound exercises, namely, give you the biggest bang for your buck as they engage multiple muscles simultaneously yielding efficient and time-saving workouts. The same is true for coristol, because when continually risen, we accumulate fat. We want to maintain muscle by limiting the amount of cortisol our bodies produce. The stress hormone can be controlled by limiting the length of our workouts to less than an hour (another reason for efficient workouts), managing stress, and sleeping 7-9 hours per night, preferably getting to bed before 11 p.m.

How Much Weight Should I Be Lifting?

Lifting heavy is a relative concept. What is heavy for you may be light for me. Heavy weights do not mean better results. Choose weights that challenge you but allow you to complete several repetitions while maintaining good form.

The optimal number of repetitions depends on whether one is looking primarily to build strength or muscle. Most people want to do both. You do that by varying the repetitions and load in some fashion, either daily or weekly. This is called undulating periodization. So if one day you're lifting heavy where your repetitions are limited to 5 then on the next training session use a weight that limits your repetitions to 10. The operative concept here is that the weight or load used is based upon how many repetitions that can be safely performed with correct form. One workout can be labeled as a high load workout, based upon the repetitions one can perform (i.e. 5 repetition max is considered high load), while the next workout could be considered a moderate load (i.e. 10 repetition max which is considered moderate load). The heavier the weight, the lower the repetitions, and vice versa.

The rest intervals, which is the rest in between sets depends on what the primary goal is as well. For strength, increase rest for 5 minutes while for increasing muscle mass limit rest intervals to no more than 3 minutes.

Varying loads and repetitions influence hormones in different ways. For example, high loads (5RM) stimulate testosterone where moderate loads (10RM) stimulate more growth hormone, both of which are effective in muscle mass and fat loss, but with slight differences in each. This is why higher repetitions are conductive to muscle mass, while lower repetitions are ideal for strength. Beyond the adaptive differences between varying loads, undulating weight and repetition is helpful because it prevents burnout. This is why I am a fan of undulating periodization.

Concerning Protein, How Much Should I Eat?

This is a tricky question to answer because it depends on the intensity of your exercise. The recommended daily allowance for protein is 0.8 grams per kilogram of weight. If you are 200 pounds, you should be consuming 80 grams of protein. Now, for one who engages in resistive exercise, you could argue that anywhere between 1.5 and 2 grams per kilogram of weight would be adequate. Research shows that when you're engaging in regular resistive exercise, it's important to consume more protein, mainly because protein forms the building blocks that will repair damaged muscles. That's critical to understand on a fundamental level when we're exercising, because that's essentially what we're doing—breaking down muscle tissue. This process illustrates the magnificence of the human body and its highly adaptive nature.

When we damage tissue, our bodies perceive that as physical stress. The body reacts to distress by wanting to adapt to it so that a future encounter with these circumstances doesn't cause a breakdown. The body adapts by getting bigger and stronger, and that's when we see muscle development.

There are many forms of proteins. But in short, proteins are essential to physical fitness because of how they elevate our metabolism and satiates our appetites. Soy protein is less desirable because researchers have found that it is linked with elevating estrogen, which is something that you want to avoid, particularly as a man. As a woman, you also want to monitor your soy intake to control hormonal influences.

Working out and eating this way provides you with the cornerstones of fitness and overall health. Many people have their hormonal dynamics in terrifying disarray, and the appropriate workout regime combined with smart protein intake can help bring them back in line. I often hear people say "I want to build muscle." But that's sometimes difficult to achieve.

Most people don't realize the inner workings of the body or the strategy that goes into bodybuilding. If you look at bodybuilders, for example, they have off-seasons. During these months, they're bulking up and gaining fat along the way. Come competition time, they start slimming down. By filling out muscle-wise in the off-season, they can sculpt down as they prepare for competitions. This process of optimizing muscle growth requires a high calorie and protein diet with calories consumed being 500-1000 calories greater than what they're expending on a daily basis. This is what allows them to maximize muscle growth. But if you're not looking to gain fat and you're solely concerned with optimizing muscle growth, you want to plan for a high protein and fat diet, along with high resistive exercise.

The National Strength and Conditioning Association says that a high-calorie diet joined with a compound base training program will force the highest levels of spring gain and muscle development. While protein and calories are important to consider, there are many other nutrients at play that contribute to the transformative process. Furthermore, it would be safe to say that most people don't want to gain fat in order to optimize muscle, which is why fat should be increased and carbohydrates should be decreased. Currently, there are many diets that are evidence-based and effective in accomplishing this. Paleo, ketogenic, Bulletproof and Whole30 are some of them. While they each have there distinctive features, they all function in a similar template. That is, they eliminate processed foods, high fructose corn syrup, hydrogenated fats and focus on the consumption of healthy fats and quality protein sources.

Whatever your goals, it's important to understand how your body responds to different types of exercise and what type of diet best suits your goals and physiology.

CHAPTER EIGHT

Take Control of Your Business

"Your business is a reflection of the organization within your life."

— Dr. Ivan Hernandez

They say that beauty is skin deep, and the same is true for health and business. I came to this vivid realization after my heart attack. What we see on the outside and what is present on the inside may in fact be antithetical realities. Although my business appeared to be thriving, it had become deeply strained. The volume of my clientele indicated a robust, successful company, but the rapid growth and lack of reliable employees destabilized the organization. Aside from Tee, I didn't have a business partner on whom I could rely. Worst of all, the personal guarantee I had signed to secure my second location had exposed the business and my family to failure and hardship.

No matter how much I was doing right in terms of exercising and eating well, my emotional and professional lives were under such strain that they counteracted any progress I was making. My world began crumbling due to the lack of mental wellness. What happened to me was the cumulative effect of years of tension and worry, which became intolerable by the time of my heart attack. There was an exponential increase in the dysfunction and distress, and the combination led to the almost fatal episode. When it comes to health, we must go deeper than appearance. Just because someone seems healthy on the outside does not mean he or she is absent of diseases. Just because there is no diagnosis or apparent problem doesn't mean one does not exist. Issues can brew on a micro level over time. Subtle internal changes can manifest into something sinister and damaging.

My Business Affairs

What one thinks of as coincidence may simply be the interconnectedness of luck. There's an emotional fog that often impedes decision-making in all realms of life, including personal, professional, and even spiritual circumstances. In retrospect, I have 20/20 vision. I look back on the circumstances precipitating my heart attack and know that everything was meant to happen as it did. Back then, I believed I was suffering from a run of bad luck. From my ex's increased distance and cheating to filing Chapter 11 on my business, everything fell apart at once. Certainly, those were not the best of times. Never could I have imagined back then that my life would take the direction it did. But I realize now that there was something linking all of these events.

By the time I had a heart attack, I had gotten myself into a position where I didn't have peace of mind. I was not healthy, and therefore I made mistakes. I wasn't functioning at my potential because I was not addressing my mental state. There were many things I could have addressed differently, and I see those missed opportunities now. But I was in a broken down space and the only person who knew or could treat it was me. To others, I looked perfectly healthy, just a guy with some business and personal problems I was sorting out.

I disregarded the interconnectedness of wellness and all the other dimensions that were so important. Now I ask myself, was it bad luck? Or was I exacerbating these events by being unequipped to see them clearly due to my stressed mental state? I wasn't prepared to make executive-level decisions at the time.

I was under extreme stress, and the problems from my personal life spilled over into my professional sphere. The longer this vicious cycle of problems went unresolved, the more it wore away at me mentally. While I was physically active and taking care of myself, I was weak and depleted inside. My mind was festering, bruised, and beaten from the endless emotional roller coaster. Rather than stepping back to treat the wounds, I kept hanging on for another ride.

So I'll say it again: The mind, body, and spirit are interconnected. If one suffers, it will take the others out, no matter how much energy and attention you invest in these areas individually. We have to monitor and nurture all three to be truly healthy.

When you go through hardship, it is like a puzzle, and you become a detective. You are constantly searching for the underlying cause. People go to a doctor because they are looking for what is causing their pain. The same methodology should apply to life in general. When we have pain, it is usually a manifestation of something that's happening elsewhere. When my body broke down, it was a result of my poor mental health. Unfortunately, I didn't identify the issue until after I nearly died. However, once I identified it, I was able to make changes to my life that eliminated the adverse effects on my mental state. In some cases, I simply had to make a decision and stick to it, no matter how difficult it was.

After years of bitterness and heartbreak, I finally let my ex go. She and I now communicate only with regard to the children. I assessed my other relationships as well. Painful though it was, I disengaged from friends who brought negative energy into my life. There were too many people who left me feeling drained and unhappy every time we saw one another. That part was challenging, and I missed some of those people. But I was mentally healthier, and I could not sacrifice that.

I began to see my life circumstances less in terms of good or bad luck and more through the lens of good and bad energy. Each of us possesses a limited supply of energy, so you have to channel it in the right direction. Channeling energy into people and projects that are of a positive nature will result in good "luck," or happy coincidences, however you choose to see it.

We need to take a step back and do some introspection and psychoanalysis and try to understand who we are, what our pitfalls are, and why we are susceptible to them. If you can identify these things, you can begin to rectify areas that need improvement. Then you'll find that you're filled with a positive energy that will be reciprocated the more you embody it in your life. After taking stock of my relationships and preserving only those that were uplifting, I found that I was fortunate enough to be surrounded by a good number of positive people. In many ways, I feel like I've hit the lottery in the year and a half since my heart attack. The people with whom I have deepened my connections and those I have met following my recovery are astounding human beings who have helped me turn my life around.

Ultimately, I think real health is about identifying your weaknesses and cultivating the right energy. Not everyone struggles with mental health challenges, but we all have burdens we must carry and demons we must conquer. It's up to each of us to find the root causes of our misfortunes or unhappiness and seek to correct them. For instance, some people believe that Americans are generally inactive because we overeat and therefore gain weight. Eventually, we become so big that we don't want to move, perpetuating the problem. But the opposite is true. Many Americans live unhealthy, sedentary lifestyles in which we get little movement. We become reluctant to exercise and avoid even simple activities, such as walking to the store. Why walk anywhere when there are ride companies that offer door-to-door service? Everything is accessible, and everything can be conveniently delivered without us ever needing to move. While technology brings tremendous progress, it also has detrimental side effects that contribute to widespread health problems. Each of us must be willing to take a deep look into our own circumstances to determine which misconceptions we have allowed to govern our lives and how we can free ourselves from these negative patterns.

Overcoming the inevitable obstacles and hardships that we encounter in this human experience and seeking joy every day are not easy things to do. Finding the right people to help us achieve these goals and join us on the journey is a blessing.

Despite the challenges I endured with the lawsuit, I don't regret the business decisions that I made. While there were variables that were beyond my control, I can still tip my hat to the fact that I was able to take a risk. Yes, things went wrong. But I have no regrets because I learned so much through those business experiences. There's so much we can't know when undertaking a business venture. We must be willing to learn and adapt along the way. If we concede to not knowing everything and we hire and network with the right people, the process becomes easier. In time, we make fewer mistakes. Surrounding yourself with the right people helps make up for your business inadequacies. When you're uncertain about a decision, a trusted voice will step in with the expertise you need to be successful. As a business owner, you have to know that it is okay to ask for help. You must be willing to ask for and accept assistance. There are so many variables that arise when running a business, and a wise entrepreneur seeks help when he or she requires it, whether that's in marketing, management, accounting, planning, or any other area of the business.

When you're an entrepreneur especially, business and health intertwine. You can't allow your business to run your health into the ground. If you squander your health for wealth, you will face immeasurable problems in the long-term. As soon as you start making money with your business, the first priority should be investing in quality staff to help the company grow. Too often, people simply take larger salaries rather than building up their support staffs and investing in income-generating assets. They find themselves drowning after a few years because they thought they could do everything and learned the hard way that they could not. That's when it becomes very difficult to get out of the hole, because they've created unsustainable lifestyles and can't afford to hire new employees.

I made this mistake myself, and I still wish I had spent my money on income-generating assets instead of liabilities. A big house, cars, vacations—these are all fun, but they reduce cash flow. I should have considered buying the property where my business resides and should have invested more heavily in long-term benefits for the business. Had I spent a portion of the money I paid in rentals on business real estate, I could have generated more cash flow for myself and the company.

What I learned in hindsight is that you can't allow the business to run you. You should be making decisions that enable you to manage from afar without needing to be on site all the time. Think of people who own multiple stores. They created a business model, work ethic, and culture that can thrive without them being there all the time. Like me, however, many people believe that no one else can follow through on their visions and therefore try to do everything themselves, to their own detriments.

Takeaways on Business

When you go into business, you must be willing to take risks, but do so in a calculated fashion with the guidance of seasoned accountants, lawyers, and mentors.

- Take care of your home base before moving on to the next one.
- Before considering an expansion in any type of business, be confident that your existing company can operate effectively without you, as the expansion will call for a lot of your attention.
- Identify and prioritize resources appropriately.
- Human resources will be your biggest monthly expense, but it will also be your greatest asset to the solvency of your business.
- Success is the culmination of two variables: hard work and consistency.

- Grit, grind, and guidance are what your business needs to survive. You must be the skeleton of the business, the pillar of support, and the epitome of earnestness.
- With time, everything changes.

We must have the willingness and adaptability to adjust as the business and market shifts. Otherwise, we will be left behind. The variables that surrounds one's respective business are rarely fixed.

CHAPTER NINE
5 Pillars of Optimal Wellness

"Having a plan is vital to achieve any success, including optimal wellness."

— Dr. Ivan Hernandez

Many people want to embark upon a transformative process that will allow them to make the changes they know will improve their lives. A healthy mindset begins with these beliefs because thoughts dictate behavior. However, having the mindset to transform will go to waste if you don't understand the steps required to make such a metamorphosis. In this chapter, I will discuss the five pillars of optimal wellness. Each pillar is key to making a significant change in your body. These are simple, logistical takeaways you can use in your daily life to stay motivated.

It is not uncommon for people to join the gym with great zeal at the beginning of the year, with high hopes of losing weight. By the end of May, if not sooner, that zeal dissipates because people are not seeing results. They didn't make the simplistic changes necessary to optimize the weight loss journey. These five pillars keep the energy and zeal going because they teach you to make changes that impact your lifestyle outside the gym. Though these may seem like small tweaks, the following pillars can make all the difference in whether you succeed. Optimal wellness must be a part of your whole life, and you have to be completely committed to achieving the results you desire.

Mindset:

As we've learned, each of the domains that constitute wellness is interdependent. But if I had to identify the most critical dimension, I would argue that establishing the right mental state is the first priority. Without the determination and will to overcome challenges, you will have an extremely difficult time fulfilling your mission.

The right mindset is vital to successfully completing any journey. No matter what you hope to achieve, stress and discomfort are part of change. Your body will recognize these stressors and respond to stress hormones, causing painful sensations and resistance initially. However, as you continue to move forward, you will reach a point at which your body instinctively reacts to the conditions you've created. Your body moves from a state of consciousness to unconsciousness while on this path. The natural survival instincts will take over, and you will find yourself able to move forward despite any hardship. This is when you get into a flow state of mind and where you begin to enjoy the activities in which you have become immersed. You develop the resilience to manage stress, and you recognize and welcome the challenges.

Let me be clear that while I think having a mindset is one of the five pillars of optimal wellness, there is no universal definition of optimal wellness. In a general sense, I believe that this state of being involves a positive and resilient attitude. How those attributes play out depends on each person and his or her approach to wellness. We all can be optimally well and look extremely different from one another. Optimal wellness is not just about outward appearance, but rather what's beneath that glowing exterior.

It is extremely important to understand the effects of the mind on the body. This understanding is key to finding the energy that feeds the yearning for wellness. Your mind will be your biggest cheerleader or your greatest enemy, depending which impulses you indulge. If you know going into any journey that you're going to feel some resistance, you can prepare yourself for how to handle it. When we anticipate stress, we manage it better than when we allow it to take us by surprise.

Resilience is a positive side effect of being healthy, and it grows as we persevere. This attribute makes us more capable of bouncing back physically and mentally. We must sometimes enter uncharted territory. When we do this, we must suppress our egos and know that something great is waiting on the other side. Knowing and recognizing this should serve as inspiration to forge ahead and be unfettered by the intimidating circumstances that may abound in our lives. It is through difficulty that we become inspired. We must think of hurdles and obstacles as rites of passage. They allow us to become what we were destined to be, long before our futures were formed, back when we were just atoms.

Exercise

The second pillar of health is exercise. Movement is life. As mammals, we are meant to engage in locomotive activity. But the occasional trip to the gym is not enough. Human beings in the US have stopped running, walking, playing, skipping, and dancing. We've seen the adverse effects of our sedentary lifestyles in our growing waistlines and skyrocketing disease rates. Our ancestors didn't have the luxuries we enjoy today, so they were frequently in motion. Travel by foot or with animals was common, and people could not afford to lounge and slumber. They needed to move in search of food and shelter. The benefit of this was that their bodies were likely lean and strong. Modern humans have turned away from movement, and we must find ways to incorporate movement into our existences once again. Hitting the gym is a start, but we need to look at all the areas of our lives in which we are sedentary. We sit at work, in the waiting room, while eating, while driving, and while riding public transportation. The list goes on. We need to move to get the results we are looking for in our health.

Studies have shown that the detrimental effects of inactivity cannot be undone with an hour's worth of exercise. I cannot stress enough that exercise is more than going to the gym. We need to make movement a lifestyle. Any activity is better than sitting and doing nothing. There are ways to keep the movement happening in our lives. Marching in place while watching TV or standing versus sitting when riding a bus can help. We can carry the lessons from the gym into our other activities by incorporating rowing, lifting, and squatting movements throughout our days. The stronger we are, the less fat we have, so it is important to build muscle. As humans, we are designed with fundamental movement patterns. Benching, squatting, and deadlifting stimulate the hormones necessary to build muscle. Our bodies are meant to move in these ways, and that's why these exercises are so effective. The stronger we are, the better our body composition. When I am in the gym, I focus on these positions because of the systemic effects I receive from hormones being released. Squatting will improve chest and back muscles, in addition to the legs and glutes, because testosterone is not limited to one part of the body. At the end of the day, squatting and other movements release vital hormones, so you get the most from your workout when doing these movements.

Sleep

Sleep is a modifiable risk factor that is as important as the cessation of smoking. Sleep enables our bodies to undergo a repair process. There is a tremendous amount of literature that supports the necessity of sleep and correlates the lack of it with many diseases. These include cardiovascular disease, cancer, obesity, and diabetes. Sleep is a critical factor in our well-being, yet people sacrifice it to keep up with a society that moves faster all the time. The reason we often find ourselves in need of artificial stimulants, such as coffee, is that we are not functioning to our fullest capacity when we cut corners on sleep. We use energy drinks to replace what our bodies should give us after a good night's rest—energy.

Lack of sleep also impacts our hunger hormones. Oftentimes, we compromise sleep and find ourselves using food to wake our bodies up. There is a syndrome that exists called "night shift syndrome." This is where people tend to have a lack of concentration, energy, insomnia, and, in some cases, depression. When people are depressed, they may overeat to numb or compensate for the underlying distress. Moreover, they may experience an increase in cortisol, which wakes us up in the morning. When you're staying up late, your cortisol levels rise, which causes you to overeat. It's important for us, especially those who are truly night shift workers, to create regular habits. We have to focus solely on sleeping during the day and have a caveman sleeping style. This means complete darkness—no cell phone, TV, or radio. If you work a night shift job, create a nighttime environment for yourself during the day so you can trick yourself into sleeping the number of hours you need.

Periodically needing to sleep in to "catch up" on your energy levels is fine. But the pattern of not sleeping enough or at all is very dangerous. Our immune systems are at risk when we do not sleep enough. We need to understand that sleep, like lack of exercise, is a modifiable risk factor that can lead to disease.

Meditation and Stress Management

We live in a high-energy society, and our nervous systems are over-stimulated. Adults especially need to relax and slow down our nervous systems, and meditation is a great way to do that. In my career, I have treated many people who don't understand the adverse effects of not getting enough sleep and not being able to relax. We have to know how to slow ourselves down to avoid becoming overwhelmed. I have learned to step back and breathe, no matter what type of difficult situation I encounter. In through the nose and out through the mouth, one to two times at a one to two ratio (e.g., in for three seconds and out for six seconds). Focusing on your breath will help you disengage from the situation causing so much stress. Our bodies naturally become relaxed and subdued if we train them to respond to breathing practices and meditation.

Instead of allowing hardship to disrupt our sleep cycles, eating patterns, and emotional states, we need to maintain control by regulating our stress levels. For example, when arguing with someone, I have trained myself to respond in a calm speaking voice so as not to provoke the other person. This helps prevent the situation from escalating, and it keeps me calm. Stress is one of the key factors that led to the downward spiral of my health, so I am proactive about mitigating bad stress now.

Although stress is part of our daily experiences and serves an important purpose, we need to learn how to respond to its warning signals instead of brushing them off until an extreme situation occurs. The fight or flight response is in all of us and it is a survival mechanism. However, when this mechanism is on all the time, it is linked to belly fat and heightened cortisol levels. As with anything else, we must control our stress levels. By doing so, we control our health.

One way to manage stress is through meditation. Being still is something many people overlook. Settling your thoughts on a singular focus, like your breath or your chest rising and falling, helps to clear the mind. Your mind will not always be blank, but the point is to calm your mind and your nervous system.

Meditation allows us to manage our fast-paced lives. Research has shown that meditation improves stress levels, focus, and physiology. Meditation provides the perspective needed to remain mentally intact. As with all other exercise, you have to work your mind. Through meditation, I can look at my life from afar, as a third person. That perspective has helped me realize that life is good and to appreciate that I am alive. A mere five minutes of meditation every morning resets my attitude and enables me to live mindfully.

Nutrition

You are what you eat. While the quality and quantity of the foods you take in matters, timing matters equally. We live in a society where conventional wisdom has always taught us to eat small, frequent meals. While that may work for some people, I have found for myself that the 300 calories per meal I intended to eat often turns into 400 to 500 calories. Our bodies want to be satiated and when they don't feel that way, they prompt us to eat more. As a result, you eat 500-calorie meals six to eight times per day, and you gain weight. When you're regularly eating throughout the day, your body is highly dynamic, and its role is to maintain homeostasis. Therefore, when you consume food your body's goal is always to control its insulin levels.

Insulin always gets a bad rap, but it is a form of fat storage, and it has its place. The problem is that we tend to overstimulate the pancreas because we are often overeating during small meals. Since insulin is a fat source hormone, we are consistently having high-circulating free insulin caused by pancreatic overstimulation.

Many people believe the common misconception that not eating will slow down their metabolisms, which is why they fear skipping breakfast or other meals. But that logic is not entirely true, especially when you consider the types of breakfast foods we tend to eat. Common cereals, muffins, and breakfast products are often very high in sugars. You are better off eating a breakfast full of protein, or skipping the meal altogether, than consuming standard breakfast fare.

I, for one, am a proponent of intermittent daily fasting. This is when you fast for sixteen hours a day. The benefit is that all hormones begin to go into fat depleting mode. After the first three to four weeks, your body will adjust to the fasting and begin to show results.

I once came across the following quote from Viktor E. Frankl in *Man's Search for Meaning*, and it resonated with me on these topics:

> *"Man does not simply exist but always decides what his existence will become the next moment; and by the same token every human being has the freedom to change at any instant."*

That is how I approach life. We have been given free will by some supreme power. To me, we should use that gift to take mindful actions and to cultivate a greater awareness of what our choices are to make better decisions and ultimately live better lives.

That is why I decided to write this book. After surviving a lawsuit, a custody battle, the breakup of a marriage, and a heart attack, all in the span of twelve months, I realized how crucial it is that we live mindfully and with awareness of our decisions. Oftentimes we feel overwhelmed by the adversities of life, but I can tell you from personal experience that we can overcome even the harshest challenges.

Life without obstacles is merely existence. Living constitutes the ups and downs that life will bring and we have to know how to manage those low moments. One of my favorite principles is that the obstacle is the path. The wisdom in this is that we must confront that which is most troublesome to us. If we choose to walk away from adversity, we are not allowing ourselves to move forward.

Don't fear the obstacles, whether you're finalizing a divorce or closing a business. Push through the fear and persevere toward greatness. I was able to capitalize off everything that happened to me, good and bad, to develop a better version of myself. Most importantly, maintain a sound mind and stay in tune with your emotions. When you're able to remain calm in any situation, the rational, right-thinking side of you will always prevail.

Your Personal Path

Everyone's path toward optimal self-fulfillment is different. That which is a struggle for me may be a walk in the park for someone else. We must learn not to compare our paths with others' journeys. Whatever you are dealing with, know that it's okay to struggle and that you'll get through if you keep moving forward and take care of yourself. My own troubles taught me to focus on those things I can control. Concerning yourself with things that are out of your hands is a waste of time and happiness. Remember that you will make mistakes. But when they happen, never lose sight of your inner truth. Continue fighting for the future you desire, owning your failures as much as you own your wins. By admitting to failure and adjusting the path when necessary, you'll stay on the course to optimal wellness.

Final Afterword

I hope you found this book informative. It is a compilation of the antidotes and signs that transformed my life. My hope is that some of these principles can be applied to your life and will help you overcome some of your own adversities. I want to thank everyone who helped me along the way and God for providing me the insight, perseverance, and resilience to write this book while creating a legacy of which I can be proud. Most importantly, I hope this book is something my children and their children can share, enjoy, and learn from for years to come. Thank you all, and may your lives be blessed with happiness.

DR. IVAN'S QUICK TIPS

Top Health Tips

- Establish the right mindset to persevere and embark on your wellness journey.
- Remember that when your life is in balance, you experience the synergistic nature of mind, body, and spirit.
- You are what you eat.

Top Stress Buster Tips

- Recognize the profound effects of exercise and what it does to combat stress.
- Maintain a proper diet.
- Develop stress management strategies.
- Self-actualize through positive thinking and a supportive community.

DR. IVAN'S FAVORITE AFFIRMATIONS FOR SURMOUNTING LIFE'S ADVERSITIES BOLDLY

You reach your highest levels of self when you've fulfilled your most fundamental needs: shelter, food, and love. But you also need a healthy mind to achieve and sustain these elements. Affirmations can help you think positively even as stress begins to rise. Here are some of the thought processes that keep me mentally grounded.

The only constant in life is change.

I remind myself that change and adversity, as well as trials and tribulations, come with the experience of being human—and we can't escape the human experience. The human body is built to adapt and it has the ability to persevere through anything. We have to recognize our inner abilities and adapt to our environments.

We have to change. Ask yourself, who you are at work? And who are you at home? How many hats do you wear and how quickly can you evolve and adapt to those changes and be successful at those jobs? All we have to do is recognize and harness our own capabilities and adapt to new environments. When we take chances and face our fears and weaknesses, they eventually become our greatest strengths.

"Eat the frog."—Mark Twain

Tackle your most dreaded tasks before doing anything else. This is the simplest and most effective way to get past problems. Everything that comes after will seem much easier.

Remember nothing lasts forever.

Depending on the perspective one takes, one can see this as an optimistic or pessimistic adage. Growing up, my mother always reminded me of this saying, particularly during hard times. What I came away with is that even during our most formidable trials, the only panacea that exists is the passage of time.

Life's too short to wake up with regrets.

Examined in hindsight, life is both clear in its perspective and short in its duration. Therefore, I advocate taking chances in life. Of course, these risks must be calculated. You can't spend your life in a bubble. We learn through our mistakes and vicissitudes, and whether we realize it or not, we inspire and empower others to model our bold behavior. Thinking that we are not good enough, or smart enough, or prepared enough are the beliefs that cause us to avoid risks and accrue regrets. Even when I look back on my failures, I am proud of the ventures I have pursued.

Love the people who treat you right, and forget about the ones who don't.

Every day that we wake up is a precious opportunity to press the reset button. We start anew to seize the day but are not granted tomorrow by any means. We must prioritize the people who matter, paying no mind to those who bring us down. Life is too precious to waste time on negativity.

"If you get a chance, take it; if it changes your life, let it."—Bob Marley

Most opportunities arise once in a lifetime. When we see them, we must seize them. It's not uncommon for fear and apprehension to immobilize someone's progress. When we over-analyze, we paralyze ourselves and we spend the rest of our lives wondering "What if?"

Your social circle may get smaller, but your vision will grow larger.

Like a tree, we must always stand tall, growing from our roots and enjoying the view. As we mature, sometimes the landscape changes. Our desires, friends, and principles will evolve as we do. When this happens, we must remain confident in the purity of our visions, allowing our values to expand and change the farther out we are able to see.

YOUR 30-DAY
TRANSFORMATION DIARY

I have offered you my experience and expertise with the goal of enabling you to draw inspiration, make informed decisions, and transform your life. This book is meant to serve as an encouragement to those who feel stuck, complacent, set back, or unsure of how to move forward from adversity. It's for anyone who needs a little guidance and solidarity on this journey through the human experience. Trust that it is normal to fear the unknown, but with blind faith and the conviction to succeed, we conjure hope and harness the courage to continue.

Now it is up to you to take bold steps toward transforming your life. For the next thirty days, track your habits around mindset, exercise, nutrition, stress management, and sleep. I can firmly say from experiential knowledge that with diligence and consistency, you can progress toward any goal if you keep at it for thirty days. Once you create and reinforce a new habit, it will become a non-negotiable part of your wellness routine.

DAY 1

My daily affirmation:

_____

_____

What type of exercise I did today:

_____

_____

What I ate today:

_____

How many hours I slept last night and quality of sleep:

_____

_____

How I prevented or coped with stress:

_____

_____

DAY 2

My daily affirmation:

_____

_____

What type of exercise I did today:

_____

_____

What I ate today:

_____

How many hours I slept last night and quality of sleep:

_____

_____

How I prevented or coped with stress:

_____

_____

DAY 3

My daily affirmation:

_____

_____

What type of exercise I did today:

_____

_____

What I ate today:

_____

How many hours I slept last night and quality of sleep:

_____

_____

How I prevented or coped with stress:

_____

_____

DAY 4

My daily affirmation:

_____

_____

What type of exercise I did today:

_____

_____

What I ate today:

_____

How many hours I slept last night and quality of sleep:

_____

_____

How I prevented or coped with stress:

_____

_____

DAY 5

My daily affirmation:

_____

_____

What type of exercise I did today:

_____

_____

What I ate today:

_____

How many hours I slept last night and quality of sleep:

_____

_____

How I prevented or coped with stress:

_____

_____

DAY 6

My daily affirmation:

_____

_____

What type of exercise I did today:

_____

_____

What I ate today:

_____

How many hours I slept last night and quality of sleep:

_____

_____

How I prevented or coped with stress:

_____

_____

Dr. Ivan Hernandez

DAY 7

My daily affirmation:

_____

_____

What type of exercise I did today:

_____

_____

What I ate today:

_____

How many hours I slept last night and quality of sleep:

_____

_____

How I prevented or coped with stress:

_____

_____

DAY 8

My daily affirmation:

_____

_____

What type of exercise I did today:

_____

_____

What I ate today:

_____

How many hours I slept last night and quality of sleep:

_____

_____

How I prevented or coped with stress:

_____

_____

DAY 9

My daily affirmation:

_____

_____

What type of exercise I did today:

_____

_____

What I ate today:

_____

How many hours I slept last night and quality of sleep:

_____

_____

How I prevented or coped with stress:

_____

_____

DAY 10

My daily affirmation:

_____

_____

What type of exercise I did today:

_____

_____

What I ate today:

_____

How many hours I slept last night and quality of sleep:

_____

_____

How I prevented or coped with stress:

_____

_____

DAY 11

My daily affirmation:

_____

_____

What type of exercise I did today:

_____

_____

What I ate today:

_____

How many hours I slept last night and quality of sleep:

_____

_____

How I prevented or coped with stress:

_____

_____

DAY 12

My daily affirmation:

_____

_____

What type of exercise I did today:

_____

_____

What I ate today:

_____

How many hours I slept last night and quality of sleep:

_____

_____

How I prevented or coped with stress:

_____

_____

DAY 13

My daily affirmation:

_____

_____

What type of exercise I did today:

_____

_____

What I ate today:

_____

How many hours I slept last night and quality of sleep:

_____

_____

How I prevented or coped with stress:

_____

_____

DAY 14

My daily affirmation:

_____

_____

What type of exercise I did today:

_____

_____

What I ate today:

_____

How many hours I slept last night and quality of sleep:

_____

_____

How I prevented or coped with stress:

_____

_____

DAY 15

My daily affirmation:

_____

_____

What type of exercise I did today:

_____

_____

What I ate today:

_____

How many hours I slept last night and quality of sleep:

_____

_____

How I prevented or coped with stress:

_____

_____

DAY 16

My daily affirmation:

_____

_____

What type of exercise I did today:

_____

_____

What I ate today:

_____

How many hours I slept last night and quality of sleep:

_____

_____

How I prevented or coped with stress:

_____

_____

DAY 17

My daily affirmation:

_____

_____

What type of exercise I did today:

_____

_____

What I ate today:

_____

How many hours I slept last night and quality of sleep:

_____

_____

How I prevented or coped with stress:

_____

_____

DAY 18

My daily affirmation:

_____

_____

What type of exercise I did today:

_____

_____

What I ate today:

_____

How many hours I slept last night and quality of sleep:

_____

_____

How I prevented or coped with stress:

_____

_____

DAY 19

My daily affirmation:

_____

_____

What type of exercise I did today:

_____

_____

What I ate today:

_____

How many hours I slept last night and quality of sleep:

_____

_____

How I prevented or coped with stress:

_____

_____

DAY 20

My daily affirmation:

_____

_____

What type of exercise I did today:

_____

_____

What I ate today:

_____

How many hours I slept last night and quality of sleep:

_____

_____

How I prevented or coped with stress:

_____

_____

DAY 21

My daily affirmation:

_____

_____

What type of exercise I did today:

_____

_____

What I ate today:

_____

How many hours I slept last night and quality of sleep:

_____

_____

How I prevented or coped with stress:

_____

_____

DAY 22

My daily affirmation:

_____

_____

What type of exercise I did today:

_____

_____

What I ate today:

_____

How many hours I slept last night and quality of sleep:

_____

_____

How I prevented or coped with stress:

_____

_____

DAY 23

My daily affirmation:

_____

_____

What type of exercise I did today:

_____

_____

What I ate today:

_____

How many hours I slept last night and quality of sleep:

_____

_____

How I prevented or coped with stress:

_____

_____

DAY 24

My daily affirmation:

_____

_____

What type of exercise I did today:

_____

_____

What I ate today:

_____

*How many hours I slept last night and
quality of sleep:*

_____

_____

How I prevented or coped with stress:

_____

_____

DAY 25

My daily affirmation:

_____

_____

What type of exercise I did today:

_____

_____

What I ate today:

_____

How many hours I slept last night and quality of sleep:

_____

_____

How I prevented or coped with stress:

_____

_____

DAY 26

My daily affirmation:

_____

_____

What type of exercise I did today:

_____

_____

What I ate today:

_____

How many hours I slept last night and quality of sleep:

_____

_____

How I prevented or coped with stress:

_____

_____

DAY 27

My daily affirmation:

_____

_____

What type of exercise I did today:

_____

_____

What I ate today:

_____

How many hours I slept last night and quality of sleep:

_____

_____

How I prevented or coped with stress:

_____

_____

DAY 28

My daily affirmation:

_____

_____

What type of exercise I did today:

_____

_____

What I ate today:

_____

How many hours I slept last night and quality of sleep:

_____

_____

How I prevented or coped with stress:

_____

_____

DAY 29

My daily affirmation:

_____

_____

What type of exercise I did today:

_____

_____

What I ate today:

_____

How many hours I slept last night and quality of sleep:

_____

_____

How I prevented or coped with stress:

_____

_____

DAY 30

My daily affirmation:

_____

_____

What type of exercise I did today:

_____

_____

What I ate today:

_____

How many hours I slept last night and quality of sleep:

_____

_____

How I prevented or coped with stress:

_____

_____

Author's Note

Dr. Ivan Hernandez delivers an astounding account of recovering from personal adversities. The book gives readers a detailed description of how he handled betrayal, a health scare, business woes, and his body image as he evolved over the last few years. Dispelling the myth that men lack emotional intelligence, Dr. Ivan is in touch with everything that has changed his life. As he reflects on his human experience, he highlights the differences each change made on his experiences as a father, a son, and a significant other. In every battle he fought, he used the outcome to create positive change in his life. Dr. Ivan provides readers with the recipe he used for success so they can apply his approach of connecting mind, body, and spirit in their own lives. His account of what it takes to improve both physically and mentally is bold and honest.

CPSIA information can be obtained
at www.ICGtesting.com
Printed in the USA
BVOW03*1326140417
481326BV00001B/1/P

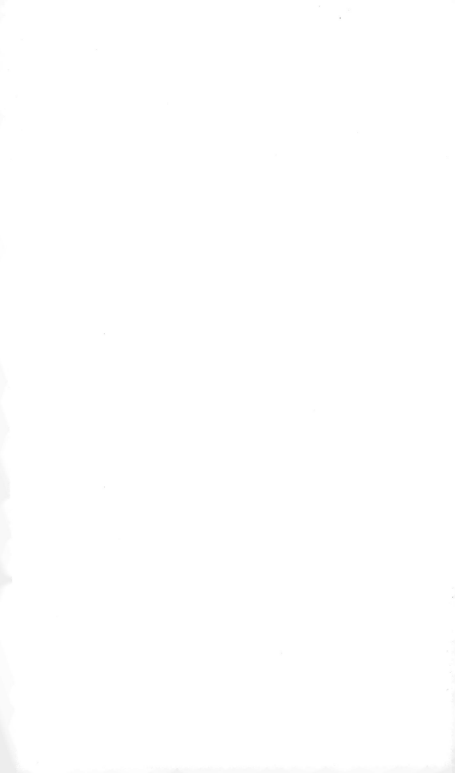